PREGNANCY

MEDICAL HELPS FOR AN EXPECTING MOTHER

DR. J. WALLER

1

Contents

INTRODUCTION

A woman's life is profoundly and dramatically changed during pregnancy, as she develops and nurtures a new life inside her body. The union of an egg and sperm results in a fertilized embryo that eventually grows into a fetus, and this is a complicated biological process. Pregnancy, which lasts for around 40 weeks, is split into three trimesters, each of which has unique phases of fetal development and changes in the mother.

When an egg and sperm fertilize each other in the fallopian tube, a zygote is created, marking the beginning of the trip. The early phases of pregnancy are then started when this fertilized egg descends the fallopian tube and inserts itself inside the uterus.

The growing fetus experiences major changes throughout the course of the three trimesters, including the development of complex systems and the establishment of basic organs and structures. The expectant mother goes through a plethora of physical and hormonal changes at the same time in order to support and care for the growing child.

Along with the obvious physical changes that occur with the expanding baby bump, pregnancy is frequently accompanied by a variety of symptoms, such as morning sickness, exhaustion, and mood swings. The health and wellbeing of the mother and the unborn child are greatly dependent on prenatal care, which includes routine checkups, ultrasounds, and any required medical operations.

Pregnancy is an emotional time of excitement and expectation, mixed with occasional difficulties. A loving home and labor and delivery plan are just two of the many things expectant parents do to get ready for the arrival of their child.

The transforming process of delivery, which delivers the baby into the world, signifies the end of a pregnancy. Giving birth can take several forms, depending on the situation. Natural childbirth, epidural, and cesarean section are among the alternatives available during labor and delivery.

The journey of pregnancy is dynamic and intensely personal, involving not just physical changes but also emotional and psychological shifts. After birth, a lifetime relationship is built on the bond between the developing baby and the expectant parents. Every pregnancy experience is unique, whether it's the first or a subsequent one, bringing with it fresh insights and happy moments as a new life is brought into the world.

CHAPTER ONE

Each of the three trimesters that make up a pregnancy lasts roughly three months, and each stage is distinguished by distinct fetal development and changes in the mother. The three phases of pregnancy are summarized as follows:

Weeks 1–12 of the first trimester:

The process of conception involves the fertilization of an egg by a sperm, resulting in the formation of a zygote. After then, the zygote divides several times in its cell before implanting into the lining of the uterus as it passes through the fallopian tube.

Embryonic Development: The embryo develops quickly in the initial several weeks. The basic structures of the main organs and systems start to take shape, and the neural tube which will eventually develop into the brain and spinal cord forms.

Major Organ Formation: By the time the first trimester ends, the heart, brain, lungs, and digestive system have all begun to take shape. We now refer to the embryo as a fetus.

Changes That Can Be Seen: Although the pregnancy may not be clearly visible, some women do suffer symptoms like weariness, breast tenderness, morning sickness, and frequent urination.

Weeks 13–26 of the second trimester:

Organ Development: In the second trimester, attention turns to the development and maturity of the systems and organs. The fetus starts to move, and fingers and toes sprout.

Visible Bump: As the baby bump grows in size, many expectant mothers experience a reduction in early pregnancy symptoms including nausea.

Fetal Movement: Pregnant women frequently experience "quickening," or fetal movements, as the fetus grows more active.

Gender Reveal: An ultrasound performed during the second trimester may be able to reveal the baby's gender under some circumstances.

Weeks 27–40 of the third trimester:

Rapid Growth: The third trimester is a time of significant growth for the fetus. The infant puts on weight while their organs continue to develop.

Immune System Development: Antibodies are passed from the mother to the fetus during the immune system's development.

Birthing Position: The infant descends onto its head in preparation for delivery. Practice contractions, also known as Braxton Hicks contractions, could happen.

Worseness: As the baby gets bigger, the mother could get worse. She might have back pain, edema, and trouble falling asleep.

The "nesting" instinct is a common one for pregnant parents, which prompts them to get the house ready for the baby's arrival.

Around the conclusion of the third trimester, labor usually starts, leading to delivery. But a full-term pregnancy can last up to forty-two weeks. As the body gets ready for the birth of a new life, the phases of pregnancy are an amazing journey that are full of emotional and physical changes. A successful pregnancy and a happy delivery experience depend on routine prenatal care, well-woman exams, and contact with healthcare professionals at every step.

A variety of symptoms and common experiences accompany pregnancy, which is a singular and transforming experience. Pregnancy shares certain common features and symptoms, even though every woman's experience is unique. Here are a few typical encounters:

Symptoms of morning sickness:

During the early stages of pregnancy, nausea and vomiting, sometimes known as morning sickness, are typical symptoms. These symptoms can manifest at any time of day, despite their name.

Exhaustion:

Excessive fatigue is a typical early indicator of pregnancy. Fatigue is caused by changes in hormones, increased blood production, and the body's energy needs for fetal development.

Changes in the Breasts:

Breast sensitivity, swelling, and soreness are typical. As blood flow rises, the breasts may also get heavier and fuller.

Urinating Frequently:

Frequent urination can be caused by increased blood flow to the pelvic area and strain on the bladder, particularly in the early and late stages of pregnancy.

Variations in Appetite:

Pregnancy is often accompanied by cravings, aversions, and changes in appetite. Certain women may grow to have strong dietary preferences or aversions to particular foods.

Changes in Mood:

Hormonal changes have the potential to affect mood, resulting in elevated feelings and mood swings. Pregnancy is a common time for emotional changes.

Gained weight:

To support the growth of the fetus, the placenta, and other maternal tissues, gradual weight increase is normal throughout pregnancy.

Heartburn with Regurgitation:

The esophageal-gastric valve might relax due to hormonal fluctuations, resulting in dyspepsia and heartburn. The uterus can put pressure on the stomach as it grows.

Water Retention and Swelling:

Increased blood volume and hormonal changes that cause water retention can cause swelling, especially in the feet and ankles.

Pelvic discomfort and back pain:

Pelvic pain and back pain might be exacerbated by the extra weight gained and postural changes that occur during pregnancy.

Fetal Motion:

One major and thrilling aspect of pregnancy is feeling the baby move. During the second trimester, fetal movements usually become more noticeable.

Hicks Braxton Contractions:

Braxton Hicks contractions sometimes referred to as practice contractions, can happen in the third trimester. These contractions aid in the uterus's readying for labor.

Alterations in the Skin:

Hormonal fluctuations can have an impact on the skin, resulting in modifications including the darkening of the areolas, the development of stretch marks, and the formation of a line on the belly called the linea nigra.

Disruptions to Sleep:

Pregnancy-related sleep disturbances can be caused by hormonal changes, discomfort, and the need for frequent restroom breaks.

The Nesting Instinct:

A common occurrence among expectant parents is the nesting instinct, which is the intense desire to arrange, tidy, and furnish the nursery in anticipation of the baby's arrival.

Although these symptoms are typical, not every woman will experience them all, and the severity varies, it's important to remember that. Furthermore, particular trimesters may have more severe versions of specific symptoms. A happy pregnancy experience is a result of getting regular prenatal care, being honest with medical professionals, and leading a healthy lifestyle. Seeking advice and assurance from a healthcare expert is advised for women who are worried about particular symptoms or experiences.

To ensure the health and wellbeing of the developing baby as well as the pregnant woman during pregnancy, prenatal care is essential. To track the pregnancy's development and handle any possible problems, it entails routine medical check-ups, tests, and advice from medical specialists. Among the essential elements of prenatal care are:

Early and Frequent Examinations:

Early in a pregnancy, preferably in the first trimester, prenatal care usually starts. Regular and early examinations enable medical professionals to keep an eye on the mother's and the developing child's health.

Physical examination and health history:

Healthcare professionals learn about the mother's medical history, medications, and past pregnancies during the initial prenatal visit. To evaluate general health, a physical examination may also be performed.

Tests on Blood:

Prenatal care frequently involves blood tests to check for infections, anemia, Rh factor, and blood type. These examinations aid in locating any possible dangers or problems that can impact the pregnancy.

Exams using ultrasounds:

Ultrasound scans are used to evaluate fetal growth and anatomy, see the developing fetus, and confirm the due date. Throughout the pregnancy, several ultrasound examinations could be performed.

Tracking Blood Pressure:

Blood pressure must be regularly monitored in order to detect and treat any signs of preeclampsia or hypertension, two diseases that might interfere with pregnancy.

Keeping an eye on weight gain:

To make sure that weight increase during pregnancy stays within a healthy range, it's critical to monitor it. The number of fetuses and pre-pregnancy weight are two factors that influence the recommended weight gain.

Screening and Genetic Testing:

Genetic screening methods, including amniocentesis or non-invasive prenatal testing (NIPT), may be recommended to determine the risk of specific genetic diseases, depending on personal preferences and circumstances.

Instruction and Guidance:

Prenatal care entails counseling and education on a range of topics related to conception, labor, and delivery. Things like diet, exercise, and getting ready for labor and delivery might be included in this.

Dietary advice

Healthcare professionals provide nutritional advice, which includes food suggestions, vitamin and mineral supplements (such iron and folic acid), and handling certain dietary issues that may arise during pregnancy.

Diagnosing gestational diabetes:

As part of standard prenatal care, women are screened for gestational diabetes, a form of the disease that can develop during pregnancy. To determine blood sugar levels, this entails glucose testing.

Shots:

It may be advised to have certain vaccinations during pregnancy to protect the mother and the unborn child, such as the flu shot and the Tdap (tetanus, diphtheria, and pertussis) vaccine.

Getting Ready for Childbirth:

Prenatal care includes talking about birth plans, labor and delivery preferences, and the many pain management alternatives that are available. Potential problems and interventions are also covered.

After-partum Routine:

Conversations on postpartum care, such as mental health issues, breastfeeding assistance, and the adjustment to parenthood, may be part of prenatal treatment.

Tracking the Movement of Fetuses:

Healthcare professionals may advise expectant moms to keep an eye on the movements of their fetus in order to gauge the health of the unborn child.

Continuous Assistance and Communication:

Healthcare professionals provide continuous support, respond to inquiries, and handle any issues during pregnancy. A happy pregnancy experience requires open communication between the expecting parents and the medical staff.

Prenatal care that is routine is linked to better pregnancy outcomes and aids in the early detection and management of any potential issues. In order to improve the mother's and the baby's health and wellbeing, it gives medical professionals the chance to provide tailored advice, support, and medical interventions as needed.

Food and Well-Being Practices

To promote the health of the expectant mother and the developing baby, it is essential to maintain a healthy lifestyle during pregnancy, including appropriate nutrition and positive habits. The following are important things to keep in mind when it comes to diet and good behaviors while pregnant:

A well-rounded diet:

Eat a range of nutrient-dense, well-balanced meals in your diet. Incorporate as many fruits, vegetables, whole grains, lean meats, dairy products, and dairy substitutes into your meals as possible.

Prenatal vitamins and folic acid:

Prior to being pregnant, begin taking folic acid-containing prenatal vitamins, and keep taking them all the way through. Folic acid protects developing babies from neural tube problems.

Proper Hydration:

Drink lots of water to stay hydrated throughout the day. Drinking enough water supports several body processes and can ease some of the discomforts associated with pregnancy.

Avoid Alcohol and Limit Caffeine:

When pregnant, cut back on caffeine and stay away from alcohol. Elevated intake of coffee has been linked to a higher chance of preterm birth, and alcohol can negatively impact the growing fetus.

Control your weight gain:

Based on your BMI prior to becoming pregnant, track your weight gain within the advised range. Inadequate weight gain may have an impact on fetal growth, whilst excessive weight gain may lead to difficulties.

CHAPTER TWO

Little Meals Often:

To control nausea and avoid overindulging, eat little, frequent meals. This strategy can assist in preserving stable blood sugar levels.

Fish Oils (Omega-3):

Incorporate omega-3 fatty acid sources into your diet, such as walnuts, chia seeds, flaxseeds, and fatty seafood (like salmon). For the development of the fetus's brain and eyes, omega-3s are crucial.

Foods High in Iron:

In order to avoid anemia, which is a typical pregnancy problem, eat meals high in iron. Dark leafy greens, lean meats, beans, lentils, and fortified cereals are all excellent sources.

Consumption of calcium:

For the baby's bones and teeth to develop properly, make sure they are getting enough calcium. Leafy greens, fortified plant-based milk, and dairy products are excellent sources of calcium.

Rich in Fiber Foods:

To encourage regular bowel movements and ward off constipation, include foods high in fiber, such as whole grains, fruits, vegetables, and legumes.

Sources of protein:

Incorporate a range of protein sources, including dairy, tofu, eggs, fish, poultry, legumes, and nuts, as well as lean meats. For a newborn to grow and thrive, protein is necessary.

Work Out Frequently:

With your doctor's permission, partake in moderate-intensity physical activities like swimming, walking, or prenatal yoga. Frequent exercise can enhance general wellbeing, help with weight management, and lower stress.

Apply Stress Reduction Techniques:

Use methods to reduce stress, such mindfulness, meditation, or deep breathing. Both the mother and the child may be affected by ongoing stress.

Get Enough Rest:

Make it a priority to get enough sleep, and create a regular sleep schedule. For general health and wellbeing throughout pregnancy, getting enough sleep is crucial.

Steer clear of undercooked or raw foods:

Steer clear of raw or undercooked meats, eggs, and shellfish to reduce your risk of contracting a foodborne illness. Maintain good hygiene and food handling practices as well.

Frequent check-ups for pregnancy:

To keep an eye on your health and handle any concerns, schedule routine prenatal checkups. During these appointments, talk to your healthcare practitioner about your dietary and lifestyle choices.

Noting that every person's nutritional demands are different, pregnant women should speak with their healthcare providers to develop a customized plan that takes into account their unique needs, dietary choices, and state of health. A happy pregnancy experience is a result of making educated nutritional decisions and forming healthy habits, which also set the groundwork for the unborn child's growth and health.

Common Questions and Difficulties

Although many pregnancies go forward without significant issues, it's crucial to be aware of typical worries and potential problems that can occur. Monitoring and resolving these concerns require regular prenatal care and open contact with healthcare practitioners. Here are a few typical pregnancy-related worries and issues:

Symptoms of morning sickness:

During the first trimester, nausea and vomiting, sometimes known as morning sickness, can happen. It might continue during pregnancy in certain situations.

Diabetes During Gestation:

Pregnancy can cause a kind of diabetes called gestational diabetes, which affects some women. Diet, exercise, and occasionally medication can help manage it.

Pre-eclampsia:

High blood pressure and organ damage are the hallmarks of preeclampsia, which usually develops after 20 weeks of pregnancy. To identify preeclampsia symptoms, routine blood pressure monitoring is essential.

Early Labor:

The phrase "preterm labor" describes labor that begins before 37 weeks of gestation. Premature birth may arise from it, and the baby may experience problems.

Anemia:

Pregnancy is frequently associated with anemia, a disorder marked by a low red blood cell count. Foods high in iron and iron supplements are frequently advised.

infections of the urinary tract (UTIs):

Women who are expecting have a higher risk of UTIs. Treatment must begin right away in order to avoid problems.

Pregnancy loss:

A miscarriage is when a pregnancy ends before 20 weeks. There are several possible causes for this. Early pregnancy monitoring and care can assist in identifying and resolving possible problems.

Unwanted Pregnancy:

Fertilized eggs that implant outside of the uterus—typically in the fallopian tube—cause an ectopic pregnancy. This can be quite dangerous and has to be treated medically right away.

Previa Placenta:

When the placenta covers the cervix entirely or partially, it is known as placenta previa. To avoid problems, changes to the birth plan can be necessary.

Contamination by Group B Streptococcus (GBS):

Some women carry the bacteria known as GBS without experiencing any symptoms. During labor, it may be transferred to the infant and result in infection. It is common for carriers to be advised to take antibiotics during childbirth.

Rh Non-Compatibility:

When a baby is Rh-positive and the mother is Rh-negative, Rh incompatibility may result. In order to avoid problems in future pregnancies, Rh immunoglobulin is given.

Growth Restriction Within the Uterus (IUGR):

When a baby does not develop in the uterus at the anticipated rate, it is referred to as IUGR. It can result in low birth weight and be linked to a number of different things.

Multiple Gestation: (e.g., twins, triplets)

There is a higher chance of difficulties with multiple gestation pregnancies, such as low birth weight, early delivery, and other difficulties.

Separating polyhydramnios from oligohydramnios

Amniotic fluid excess is known as polyhydramnios, whereas amniotic fluid deficiency is known as oligohydramnios. Intervention and monitoring may be necessary for both disorders.

Inadequate Nervous System:

Premature birth is more likely in cases of cervical insufficiency, which is characterized by the cervix opening prematurely during pregnancy. Cervical cerclage is one possible treatment for it.

It's crucial to remember that every person's experience is unique and that this is not an entire list. Early detection via routine prenatal exams, conversation with healthcare practitioners, and adherence to suggested guidelines and remedies are crucial for managing issues and difficulties. Any unexpected symptoms or concerns should be reported right away by pregnant patients to their healthcare team so that they can be properly evaluated and managed.

Psychological Health

A good and happy pregnancy experience is largely dependent on one's emotional wellness. Many emotions are experienced throughout pregnancy, and it is crucial for expectant mothers to take care of their mental and emotional needs as well as the developing baby's health. The following are some methods to help with emotional health during pregnancy:

Honest Communication:

Share your thoughts, worries, and expectations in an honest and open manner with your significant other, family, and friends. Create a network of support by sharing the pleasures and difficulties of pregnancy.

Antenatal Education

Attend educational workshops and prenatal classes to gain more knowledge about the changes that occur throughout pregnancy, labor, and the postpartum period. Being informed can empower one and reduce anxiety.

Frequent check-ups for pregnancy:

Keep an eye on your physical and mental health by scheduling routine pregnancy checkups. Talk to your healthcare professional about any emotional issues you may have.

Create a Support Network:

Embrace the network of friends and relatives who will always be there for you. Talk about your experiences, ask for guidance, and rely on your network of support as required.

Practices of Self-Care:

Make relaxing and joyful self-care activities a priority. This can involve reading, going on walks, engaging in mindfulness exercises, or pursuing hobbies.

Healthy Living Options:

Consume a diet rich in nutrients, undertake regular exercise (as directed by your healthcare professional), and get enough sleep to maintain a healthy lifestyle.

Accept Modifications:

The emotional and physical changes that accompany pregnancy should be welcomed and accepted. Remember that it's okay to feel a variety of emotions, and practice self-compassion.

Meditation and mindfulness:

To stay present and lower stress, engage in mindfulness and meditation practices. Methods like guided visualization and deep breathing have their uses.

Describe Your Emotions:

Use discussion, art, or journaling as a way to express your emotions. Permit yourself to investigate and comprehend your feelings.

Make a future plan:

Establish goals and objectives for the future, such as your postpartum care and delivery plan. A sense of control and less uncertainty can be gained from knowing what to expect.

Learn All You Can About Postpartum:

Discover the feelings and difficulties that come with being a new mother. Preparing for the postpartum period can be aided by knowing that postpartum feelings are normal and by seeking support when necessary.

Expert Assist:

You should think about getting professional help if you frequently feel depressed, anxious, or experiencing other mental health issues. Expert help on perinatal mental health can be obtained from a therapist or counselor with this experience.

Make Contact with Other Expectant Mothers:

To meet other expectant parents, enroll in prenatal classes or support groups. Creating relationships and exchanging experiences can foster a feeling of community.

Honor major achievements:

Celebrate and record pregnancy milestones, including the first kicks you feel or finishing a particular trimester. Make happy recollections and think back on the trip.

Establish Reasonable Expectations:

For both you and your partner, set reasonable expectations. Recognize that being a parent presents problems and that it's acceptable to ask for assistance.

Recall that every person has a different level of emotional well-being, and that experiencing a wide range of emotions is common throughout pregnancy. A happy and satisfying pregnant experience is facilitated by putting self-care first, getting help, and maintaining contact with your emotional needs. Never be afraid to seek advice and help from a mental health expert or your healthcare provider if you're feeling overwhelmed.

Getting Ready to Give Birth

To guarantee a joyful and powerful experience, preparing for childbirth entails a blend of practical, emotional, and physical aspects. As you get ready to give birth, keep the following important factors in mind:

Become Informed:

Enroll in classes on childbirth education to gain an understanding of labor phases, pain relief alternatives, and the delivery process. Making educated decisions is facilitated by knowledge.

Establish a Birth Plan:

Create a birth plan that includes your desired outcomes for the labor, delivery, and postpartum period. Talk about it with your doctor, and be willing to change your mind if necessary.

Participate in Prenatal Education:

Take part in prenatal workshops that address issues including breathing exercises, relaxation techniques, and the role of your delivery partner. These courses offer useful skills related to labor and delivery.

Keep Moving:

With the approval of your healthcare physician, start moderate-intensity exercise on a regular basis. Maintaining strength and flexibility can be aided by exercises like swimming, yoga for pregnant women, and walking.

Utilize Breathing Exercises:

To control pain and maintain attention during contractions, learn and practice different breathing techniques. Breathing deeply and rhythmically both have benefits.

Think About Pain Management Choices:

Investigate your alternatives for pain management. These include medical interventions like epidurals and complementary therapies like massage and hydrotherapy. Understand the options that are accessible to you.

Take a look around the Birthing Facility:

To become acquainted with the surroundings, get to know the personnel, and learn about the amenities offered, take a tour of the birthing center.

Assemble a Hospital Bag:

Well in advance, prepare a hospital bag. Pack necessities like cozy clothes, toiletries, snacks, crucial paperwork, and stuff for you and the infant.

Form a Birth Support Team:

Select a supportive birth team, such as your spouse, relatives, or friends. Make sure that both you and your birth partner are in agreement by talking about roles and expectations.

Use relaxation techniques:

To help you handle stress and anxiety, try some relaxation techniques like visualization and meditation. It can help to create a peaceful mental environment before giving birth.

Talk about postpartum arrangements:

Think about postpartum plans, encompassing home care arrangements, preferred feeding methods, and any obstacles. Transitioning easier if you know what to expect after giving birth.

Discover How to Take Care of Infants:

Take part in courses or classes on breastfeeding, newborn safety, and infant care. Acquiring knowledge about taking care of your newborn contributes to your confidence.

Remain Nutritious and Hydrated:

To stay energized during labor, make sure you're eating and staying hydrated well. Eat light, simple-to-digest snacks.

Labor Practice Positions:

Examine various labor and delivery positions, like squatting, walking, or using a birthing ball. Changing postures can aid in pain management and speed up the delivering process.

CHAPTER THREE

Maintain Emotional Connectivity:

Maintain an emotional bond with your significant other. Discuss any worries or anxieties you may have about giving birth, communicate honestly, and express your thoughts.

Maintain Flexibility:

Plan ahead, but also be adaptable and willing to change as circumstances demand. Being flexible helps you better manage the sometimes-unpredictable experience of childbirth.

Get Your House Ready:

Get your house ready for the new baby. Prepare the nursery, wash the baby's clothes, and make sure you have all the necessary materials.

Establish a Calm Ambience:

Make your house a relaxing place. To help you relax, try aromatherapy, relaxing music, or low lighting.

Perform Comfort Measures:

Discover and put into practice comfort techniques including using heat packs, counterpressure, and massage. During labor, they may offer relief.

Seek out Mental Assistance:

Seek for emotional assistance from loved ones, friends, or support networks. As you are ready to give birth, talking to someone about your thoughts and worries might be helpful.

Recall that each delivery experience is distinct, and it's OK to handle it whatever feels most comfortable for you. You may improve your preparedness for childbirth and welcome the journey ahead by being proactive in educating yourself, maintaining your physical and mental well-being, and creating a support network.

Afterpartum Care and Beyond

The postpartum period is an important time to attend to the physical and mental health of the newborn and the new mother. Positive postpartum experiences are influenced by continued self-care and attending to the changing needs of the family after the initial postpartum period. Key elements of postpartum care and things to think about in the time after are as follows:

Quick Postpartum Care:

Hospital Stay:

While you are in the hospital, heed the advice of the medical staff. Get assistance with recovering, caring after your newborn, and nursing.

Help on an emotional level:

Maintain your emphasis on mental health. Discuss your feelings with your significant other, your family, and your friends. If necessary, get professional assistance.

Support for Breastfeeding:

Make use of lactation consultants' advice as well as other breastfeeding support options. To improve your knowledge, enroll in breastfeeding classes before to giving delivery.

Restorative and Restorative:

Give your body space to recuperate. Observe the postpartum care instructions given by medical professionals, which should include suggestions for relaxation, exercise, and hygiene.

Handling Pain:

As advised by your healthcare professional, take prescribed or over-the-counter pain relievers to manage postpartum discomfort.

Observe Bleeding After Delivery:

Monitor lacrimation (postpartum hemorrhage). Notify your healthcare provider of any unusual bleeding or changes.

Postpartum Assessment:

Participate in the postpartum examination with your physician. Address family planning alternatives, talk about any worries, and evaluate the healing process.

Beyond the Postpartum Period

Self-Nurturing:

Maintain your self-care priorities. Make time for happy hobbies, leisure, and relaxation. Sufficient self-maintenance promotes general health.

Consumption and Hydration:

Stay hydrated and eat a balanced diet—especially if you're nursing. Think about modifying your diet if needed to suit your particular demands.

Moving About:

Restart physical exercise gradually in accordance with your doctor's advice. Think about doing exercises for the pelvic floor and core strength after giving birth.

Psychological Health:

Keep an eye on and give priority to your mental health. Support-seeking is essential as postpartum mental disorders might develop. Keep in touch with your loved ones and, if necessary, think about counseling.

Parental Assistance:

Use parenting classes, internet forums, or local groups to get support for your parenting. Create relationships with other parents by exchanging tips, experiences, and guidance.

Planning a family:

Your healthcare provider should be consulted about family planning alternatives. Take into account birth control options that fit your long-term family plans.

Sleep hygiene:

Make sure you and your child have regular, healthy sleep schedules. Establish a sleeping environment that is comfortable and follow proper sleep hygiene.

Communication between partners:

Continue to speak with your partner in an open manner. As parents, we should discuss and agree upon changes to our daily routines and duties.

Development of Children:

Be up to date on activities that are appropriate for your child's age and developmental milestones. As your infant grows and develops, cherish the times you spend together.

Typical Medical Visits:

Make time for regular checkups with the doctor for both you and your child. Ensure that your child has regular check-ups, developmental evaluations, and vaccines.

Balance between work and life:

When you resume work or go about your everyday business, strike a balance between work and life. Make childcare arrangements and let employers or support systems know what you require.

Interaction with the Community:

For social support, get involved in your community. Join playgroups, parent get-togethers, or neighborhood events to make friends and exchange stories.

Exercise After Giving Birth:

Look into postpartum fitness choices like yoga or fitness programs tailored to new moms. Exercise gradually can improve both mental and physical health.

Honor major achievements:

Honor accomplishments of all sizes and milestones. Consider your parenting experience and your family's development.

It's important to keep in mind that postpartum care is a continuous process and that tactics must be modified to accommodate the family's evolving demands. A pleasant and fulfilling postpartum experience and beyond can be achieved by seeking assistance, staying in touch with healthcare providers, and maintaining a holistic approach to well-being.

Conclusion

Pregnancy is an incredible and life-changing process that involves modifications to one's physical, mental, and way of life. From the time of conception to the delivery of a new life, every phase is characterized by excitement, expectation, and the nurturing of an ever-deepening link.

During this time, the pregnant mother experiences amazing physiological changes as her body adjusts to meet the demands of her developing child. A safe and happy pregnancy experience is facilitated by regular prenatal care, education, and support from medical professionals.

From an emotional perspective, the voyage is a mosaic of happiness, adventure, and sporadic difficulties. A happy pregnancy requires taking care of one's emotional health, keeping up a network of friends and family, and getting expert assistance when necessary.

A comprehensive plan that includes education, physical fitness, and emotional preparedness is necessary to prepare for childbirth. Being adaptable and keeping lines of communication open with medical professionals are crucial in navigating the distinct journey that every childbirth takes.

A new chapter begins with postpartum care, which requires attention to the newborn's wellbeing and the recovering new mother. A happy postpartum experience is influenced by ongoing self-care, emotional support, and a comprehensive understanding of family dynamics.

The adventure doesn't finish with the postpartum phase. It continues as the family grows. The cornerstones of a happy parenting experience are adjusting to the changing requirements of the family, maintaining communication with healthcare professionals, and creating a nurturing atmosphere.

The experience of becoming pregnant is a monument to the fortitude, love, and perseverance that characterize parenthood—celebrating victories, holding onto priceless moments, and viewing obstacles as chances for personal development. During the voyage, we come to the profound conclusion that when we bring a kid into the world, we are starting an incredible journey of nurturing, guiding, and seeing their wonderful journey.

THE END